QUICK FIX
STINKY FEET REMEDIES

NATURAL FOOT CARE FOR

BROMODOSIS

LUCY RAY

COPYRIGHT

TABLE OF CONTENTS

<u>CONCLUSION</u> ....**<u>26</u>**

INTRODUCTION

Known medically as bromodosis, stinky feet are a year-round issue. Sweaty feet, paired with wearing the same shoes every day, are the main causes. Stinky feet, like bad morning breath, are caused by bacteria accumulating on your feet throughout the day. Unlike terrible morning breath, which is frequently caused by a lack of moisture in the mouth, stinky feet become smellier when moisture is introduced. Your feet are covered in sweat glands, which offer an ideal home for bacteria as they perspire throughout the day.

Germs that cause odour flourish in dark, damp conditions, which makes your socks and shoes perfect breeding grounds. Microbes thrive in both dampness and heat, and once they've found a home in your shoes, they'll cling to your feet when you take them off. Your unsightly foot odour may be the result of your naturally sweaty feet. Sweaty feet can happen to anyone, regardless of the temperature or season. Teenagers and pregnant women, on the other hand, are more vulnerable since hormonal changes induce them to sweat more.

If you're on your feet all day, under a lot of stress, or have a medical condition called hyperhidrosis, which causes you to sweat more than usual, you're more likely to experience foot perspiration. Foot odour can also be caused by a fungal infection like athlete's foot. As perspiration emerges from the pores, bacteria on the skin break it down. As the sweat decomposes, it emits a cheesy odour. It's easy to have stinky feet now and again, but the good news is that fixing them isn't too difficult. This book would provide quick fixes for stinky feet. This is the ideal opportunity to get rid of those stinky feet.

CHAPTER ONE
GETTING RID OF SMELLY FEET

Trapped sweat is the primary cause of stinky feet. The feet have thousands of sweat glands, which produce a lot of sweat throughout the day. Sweat that gets trapped in your shoes or socks can produce a foul stench. Bromodosis, or stinky feet, is the name for this condition. Bacteria are also the cause of stinky feet. Bacteria of various types can be found on the bottoms of your feet. These bacteria feed on the sweat that your foot produce regularly. When bacteria feed on sweat, they produce an acid that creates foot odour. Smelly feet are one of the most embarrassing things to have to deal with, especially if you're going to someone else's house and won't be able to remove your shoes. If you're sick of dealing with this problem, there are a few things you can do to start working on solving it once and for all. Finding out what the cause is a good place to start, and while this may sound simple, there are a few different reasons why your feet could be stinking up the place.

The majority of odorous bacteria can be found under the nails and on toughened skin. Sweating is exacerbated by hyperhidrosis, yeast infections, and stress. Yeast infection, excessive perspiration, stress, and poor hygiene can stimulate the bacteria that causes stinky feet. Our feet used to get hot from walking on the sunbaked ground before we had shoes. They were able to cool down more effectively thanks to the abundance of sweat glands. However, when we wear shoes, sweat can accumulate, resulting in smelly feet. Shoes and socks provide the ideal habitat for perspiration and bacteria to mix, which is why appropriate hygiene is so important. You might not notice the odour at first because it's only in your shoes. However, the stink will eventually grow too strong for you and everyone else to ignore. A few of the most common causes of smelly feet are listed below in this chapter of the book.

Sweaty Feet: Sweat is produced by our bodies when they need to cool down. Millions of bacteria live on sweat and shed skin cells, making the feet a natural habitat for them. If you have excessively sweaty feet, you may have hyperhidrosis, a common condition in which the soles of your feet create more perspiration than normal. Sweaty palms are another indicator of this. This isn't technically a problem for which you should see a doctor, but working with a podiatrist for this issue could be highly beneficial if you want to get rid of your stinky feet. No matter what the temperature is, the feet sweat every day. While everyone can have stinky feet, it's estimated that 10% to 15% of the population has feet that stink more than the average. You should also avoid wearing shoes or boots for lengthy periods, as this can cause this condition. True, the moisture produced by our feet evaporates before it can attract bacteria, but wearing shoes, boots, or shocks prevents evaporation, increasing the possibilities of bacteria growth.

Stress: If you have lately faced a scenario that has caused you to be more stressed than usual, this could be the cause of your stinky feet. Sweaty feet can be caused by stress. Overworking or stressful situations not only cause acne, weight gain, and migraines, but they can also cause your feet to stink. When you're stressed, you'll sweat a lot, and if you're wearing tight shoes, you'll stink.

Poor Hygiene: When it comes to thorough and deep cleaning, feet are one of the most overlooked portions of the body, which can contribute to stinky feet. One of the most common causes of stinky feet is poor hygiene. This isn't one of the more straightforward difficulties to solve, but it's one of the most common. Try spending a little more time cleaning your feet before going to the doctor to ensure that this isn't a temporary remedy. After showering, experiment with different foot lotions to improve the smell of your feet. Bromodosis can be caused by a variety of factors, including poor hygiene. You should wash your feet regularly. It's also crucial to change your socks at least once a day. When you don't keep up with your foot cleaning routine, bacteria can grow out of control, causing bad odours or making them worse.

It's not enough to simply clean your feet. You should wash them twice a day with mild soap and moisturize them as well. Some people scrub their feet only on the tops and bottoms, ignoring the region between their toes. This is where fungal diseases can be found. When it comes to stinky feet, the problem isn't so much how much your feet sweat as it is how much sweat is trapped in your shoes. Sweat has nowhere to go if your feet are not ventilated. We're more inclined to wear heavier, warmer shoes and socks in the winter, which can reduce airflow and retain sweat, allowing bacteria to thrive. When it comes to smelly feet, the problem isn't how much sweat your feet produce; it is how much sweat is trapped in your shoes. Heat isn't the only thing that makes your feet sweat. Our feet can also sweat when we step out into the cold or when the temperature changes suddenly. Bromodosis is rather frequent, especially if you wear the same shoes every day, tighten the laces, or spend a lot of time on your feet. If you don't clean your shoes or don't expose them to enough sunshine to destroy bacteria, they will smell bad.

Hormones: Our bodies are built differently. Hormones influence how much sweat is produced by the sweat glands. That's why sweaty, stinky feet are so common among pregnant women and teenagers. Stress can cause hormones to spike, so if you're going through a stressful time, your feet may show it. That is why you should replace your shoes and socks regularly and dry your feet thoroughly with a towel before putting them on. Puberty and pregnancy might cause your feet to sweat more than usual due to hormonal changes. Hyperhidrosis is a medical disease in which patients sweat excessively regularly; the palms of their hands and soles of their feet are particularly troublesome. Hormonal changes can cause sweat glands to produce excessive sweat, resulting in stinky feet in some circumstances. Teenagers and pregnant women are especially susceptible to foot sweating due to hormonal changes. Periods and menopause can cause hormonal changes in women, which can reduce perspiration production by the body, including the skin on their feet. To avoid a yeast infection, podologists recommend not just washing your feet after showering, but also wiping your toes with a cloth.

Nutrition: What you eat can have an impact on your body's functions. What a person eats can cause general body odour, including foot odour and poor breath. Food contains nutrients that are essential for our daily life, but some of them can affect our ability to smell. Excessive consumption of foods high in sulfides and other odour-causing ingredients can cause your feet, as well as the rest of your body, to stink. Ketosis odour is a disorder that affects people who consume a lot of protein. This is influenced by the low carbohydrate intake, which boosts ketones generation. The odour of ketone is similar to that of rotten fruits. Choline and carnitine, which are processed by the body to make trimethylamine, are abundant in foods that often contain particular protein types. This substance also has a fishy stench to it. Onions, garlic, asparagus, cabbage, mustard seed, red meat, and a variety of other foods might cause body odour.

CHAPTER TWO
WHEN IS SMELLY FEET A MEDICAL PROBLEM

Each foot has up to 250,000 sweat glands, and these thousands of small glands can produce up to one pint of sweat every day. Numerous bacteria thrive in the combination of water and salt found on human feet. The bacteria that cause feet to stink are those that thrive on sweat and dead skin cells. While foot odour may not always indicate a health condition, it can be an indicator of a medical problem in some cases. Hyperhidrosis, for example, is a condition in which one's sweat glands create excessive sweat, which might result in a stench. Similarly, fungal infections, which are quite frequent, can result in dry, flaky skin, which bacteria love to feast on. Both of these problems have potential treatments, so go to your doctor if you think you could be suffering from one of them.

Foot odour can also be caused by non-medical reasons. Footwear composed of unbreathable synthetic materials can prevent sweat from evaporating, allowing bacteria to thrive in a humid atmosphere. Synthetic-fabric socks can have a similar effect. As a result, choosing footwear made of natural fibers is the greatest way to eliminate foot odours such as cotton. When it comes to foot odour, cleanliness can make a difference. Dry your feet thoroughly after showering and change your socks and shoes regularly. If the condition persists, an over-the-counter foot odour remedy may be used. In spray and powder form, there are a range of antibacterial, antifungal, and deodorizing choices that are safe, effective, and well accepted by most individuals. Smelly feet can sometimes be a sign of more serious problems. In this chapter, you'll find various cases to consider regarding the medical causes of smelly feet.

Athlete's foot: This is a fungal infection that causes the skin to crack, flake, blister, and itch. It can also cause your feet to stink. Other fungal infections, such as ringworm and jock itch, are closely related to athlete's foot. The infection can be treated with over-the-counter antifungal drugs, but it usually returns. While a continuous athlete's foot treatment strategy is necessary to eliminate the fungal foot infection, prevention is always preferable than cure. A scaly red rash is the most common symptom of athlete's foot. The rash usually appears between the toes. When you take off your shoes and socks, the itching is usually the worst. Chronic dryness and scaling on the soles of the feet that extends up the side of the foot are symptoms of athlete's foot. It's easy to confuse it with eczema or dry skin. The illness can affect one or both of your feet, it can spread to your hand if you scratch or pick at the infected areas. A scaly rash with itching, stinging, and burning are common signs and symptoms of athlete's foot. Athlete's foot is contagious and can be passed from person to person via contaminated floors, towels, or clothing.

The infection of athlete's foot can spread to other parts of the body, including the nails, groin, and hands. Scratching or picking at infected areas of the feet can lead to an infection in one or more sections of the body. Athlete's foot fungi can also infect your toenails, which are more resistant to therapy than the rest of your body, because the fungus can travel on your hands or a towel, it's typical for the infection to migrate from your feet to your crotch. If a rash on your foot persists after two weeks of self-treatment with over-the-counter antifungal medicine, see your doctor. Consult your doctor if you feel you have athlete's foot and detect any signs of a subsequent bacterial infection, such as severe redness, swelling, discharge, or fever.

Pitted keratolysis: This is a medical problem that necessitates a visit to the doctor. A common cause of smelly feet is pitted keratolysis. You might not realize you have it unless you look attentively. Pitted keratolysis is a condition in which bacteria consume the skin on the soles of the feet, causing a white pitted look and a cheesy odour. A kind of pitted keratolysis in which the damaged portions of the skin turn red is also known. The pits do not normally cause other symptoms, they can become uncomfortable or itch when pressure is applied to the foot while walking. Pitted keratolysis is a bacterial skin infection that can affect the soles of your feet as well as the palms of your hands.

Due to the sweaty environment caused by wearing shoes and socks for long period of time, this condition frequently affects the feet. Small pits in the top layer of skin and regions of white skin distinguish it. It's the cause of smelly feet, and it affects far more men than women. The little pits or indentations on the soles of the feet are normally circular and range in diameter from 0.5 to 7 millimeters. Pitted keratolysis is caused by a variety of bacteria, the most frequent of which being Actinomyces Dermatophilus, Corynebacteria congolensis, Streptomyces, and Kytococcus sedentarius. These bacteria thrive in damp or moist environments. This is why it is so common among persons who do not allow their feet to breathe enough. Protease enzymes are produced by germs on the feet or palms, which damage the epidermis' topmost layer, resulting in pitting. Sulfur chemicals produced by microorganisms on the skin are the source of the foul odour. Athletes, military members, farmers, pedicure and foot carers, fishermen, industrial workers, sailors, and other persons who are exposed to the risk of developing Pitted keratolysis are among those at risk. Pitted keratolysis is caused by the following factors: Excessive sweating of the hands and feet, diabetes, occlusive footwear such as rubber boots or vinyl shoes, immunodeficiency, thicker skin of the palms and soles, ageing, and hot and humid conditions are all causes of excessive sweating of the hands and feet.

Medication: Some drugs can cause smell in the feet. Medication has a vast number of adverse effects that can have an impact on your feet. It's possible that the pain in your feet or increased sweating you're experiencing after starting a new drug isn't a coincidence. A lot of medicines turns out to alter the human sweating response. Most of the time, this is normal, but it might also indicate something more serious. Antidepressants, heartburn and reflux medications, asthma inhalers, pain relievers, diabetes medications, breast cancer medications, anti-inflammatory drugs, and a variety of other medications can raise serotonin levels, affecting how the body regulates temperature and resulting in excessive sweating. After two or three days, doctors may ask patients to report any negative effects they are having from taking specific medications. Some injections suppress testosterone levels in males and estrogen levels in women, which can lead to night sweats and excessive sweating. Speak with your doctor if a side effect of a drug you're taking is generating an unpleasant odour. They can assist you in determining your alternatives, which may include changing your dose or switching to a different medicine.

Do not discontinue taking any medications without first consulting your doctor

CHAPTER 3
QUICK REMEDIES FOR SMELLY FEET

Foot odour, it turns out, isn't actually caused by the feet. The bacteria on the feet, as well as the filthy socks and shoes that cover them, cause the odour. Those bacteria, like us, get rid of garbage; it's the trash that stinks so terrible. After bathing, soaking, or swimming, dry your feet thoroughly using whatever method you prefer. Moisture causes unpleasant odours, so keep your feet, shoes, and socks as dry as possible. You can also keep your feet dry by wearing cotton socks and wearing shoes made of natural materials like cotton or leather. The moisture on your foot can dissipate thanks to these natural materials. Moisture is trapped in man-made materials like nylon and plastic. Toenail fungus can be avoided by keeping your toenails clipped and clean. Using a foot file, gently remove any hard skin. When skin is firm, it can become moist and soggy, providing an ideal environment for germs to thrive. Salt baths, tea soaks, and apple cider vinegar are just a few of the home cures you can try. These measures, along with regular hygiene and shoe rotation, may assist to reduce foot odour. Lavender, eucalyptus, rosemary cajuput, and camphor are antibacterial compounds that can help eliminate odours while also soothing and softening sore feet and clearing up toenail fungus.

Remedy Soap: Keeping your feet clean, and I mean truly clean, is essential for avoiding nasty foot odours. Tea tree oil, mint, and aloe vera are used in antifungal soap to fight obstinate fungal and bacterial infections that can produce stinky feet. Wash your feet at least once a day with a mild soap. Showering in the morning or evening is the optimum time to accomplish this. Ensure that dry, itchy, or irritated skin is moisturized. Use this on a daily basis to clean your feet or any other places that need to be cleaned thoroughly, such as your underarms.

Foot Care: Exfoliating your feet is an important part of your foot care routine. Exfoliation of the feet aids in the removal of dead skin cells. Bacteria thrive on dead skin cells, therefore eliminating them effectively reduces the risk of bacterial illness. Feet exfoliation should be done one to two times per week, and in severe cases of smelly feet, two to three times each week. Exfoliation of the feet can be done with a pumice stone or with natural scrubs such as a loofah, walnut shell dust, and so on. Exfoliation is a technique for removing dead skin cells from the foot. Exfoliation should be done gently so that only dead skin cells are removed and the feet do not become damaged. Effective foot exfoliation can also be achieved with a proper pedicure.

Shoe Powder: This will eliminate the bacteria that cause odours in your sneakers and make your house stink. To absorb moisture, simply sprinkle it in your shoes every day for a few days. You'll eventually get to the point where you just need to apply it once or twice a month to get rid of shoe odour. One of the simplest and most efficient home treatments for smelly feet is talcum powder. Talcum powder or baby powder, both of which are useful in eliminating the foul odour arising from feet, are found in almost every household. Talc is a clay mineral that comprises hydrated magnesium silicate and oxygen in the form of hydrated magnesium silicate. It works by absorbing excess moisture in the feet and keeping them dry for an extended period of time.

Antifungal Spray: Athlete's foot is a fungal infection that affects the skin between the toes and is commonly caused by sweaty feet. Antifungal spray gives immediate relief from the odour and itching that are common side effects of this illness. This quick-drying spray absorbs sweat, preventing bacteria, fungus, and athlete's foot on your feet.

Disinfect your shoes: You don't have to throw away your shoes if they're surrounded by a green cloud of odour even while you're not wearing them. Remove the insole from the shoe, lightly spritz it, and set it aside to dry for 24 hours. After that, you've treated the shoe by re-inserting the insole. The scent coming from your kicks may be taken care of using a general-purpose disinfectant spray like the kind you'd use in the kitchen. Look for a sanitizing kitchen spray that contains ethanol and other bacteria-killing chemicals. The longer you tolerate stinky feet, the worse the stench becomes, and even your closest friends may be unwilling to tell you the truth, so take action now. You've got nothing to lose except that odour.

CHAPTER 4
Essential Oil for Smelly Feet

One of the finest treatments for stinky feet is essential oils. Due to their potent medicinal effects, essential oils are particularly effective in removing foot odour. Essential oil has been used for antifungal, antibacterial, antiseptic, antiviral, and anesthetic purposes for decades. It's regarded as one of the most effective natural cures for stinky feet. While the name bromodosis may be frightening, stinky feet are a simple and affordable problem to solve. You might not even need to see a Podiatrist. Natural essential oils can help you get rid of even the strongest foot odours. Essential oils are known for their ability to soothe and calm. Air fresheners, candles, soaps, bath bombs, and perfumes all utilize their long-lasting aroma. Most spas utilize essential oils as one of the natural cures for smelly feet. Essential oils include antifungal, antibacterial, and antimicrobial characteristics, which help to combat germs, bacteria, fungi, and microorganisms that cause athlete's foot and nail funguses, as well as odour. Essential oils have pleasant aromas that naturally conceal unpleasant odours and replace them with a pleasant fresh scent. Some essential oils are not only antimicrobial, but they also deodorize naturally. These essential oils not only fight odour-causing germs, but they also help you reclaim your feet's healthy scent.

The absorption spots on the human foot are many. When essential oils are absorbed into those spots, they aid in the elimination of fungi, germs, and, of course, odour. Your feet are linked to many sections of your body. When you apply pressure to or touch specific portions of your feet, it might impact other parts of your body. Not to mention, using essential oils on your feet allows you to get a good night's sleep. Because your feet are the least sensitive part of your body, applying essential oils to them is generally safe. Because the feet area is not as sensitive as the arms or the face, most essential oils do not need to be diluted when applied to the foot. Soaking your feet is one of the most effective ways to improve your overall foot health and permanently eliminate foot odour. Tea tree essential oil, for example, would eradicate any unpleasant scents arising from your shoes. They love the zingy lemon eucalyptus aroma so much that they use it as an air freshener in the bathroom, kitchen, and anywhere else where a burst of freshness is needed. Keep your essential oils out of the reach of children and pets at all times. While there is no treatment for stinky feet, there are things you may do to reduce and control the odour effectively.

Lavender Essential Oil: The aroma of lavender oil is soothing and delicious, and it can put you in a light trance. The lavender plant produces lavender oil, which is an essential oil. It is one of the most powerful essential oils, with numerous health advantages. Lavender essential oil calms stress, alleviates allergy symptoms, and decreases acne. Most notably, it aids in the elimination of foot odour. Antifungal and anti-inflammatory effects are found in lavender oil. It can be used to treat eczema as well as fight microorganisms. Before going to bed, rub a few drops of lavender essential oil on your feet to kill odorous bacteria. After applying lavender to your feet, don't forget to put on your socks. Lavender oil unclogs pores and reduces inflammation when applied to the skin. Lavender oil has antibacterial and antiviral properties in addition to its pleasant aroma. Lavender oil is a well-known favourite among essential oil enthusiasts, and those who suffer from foot odour will be relieved to learn that this pleasant oil can also kill bacteria that cause odour. Lavender oil is one of the more gentle essential oils. Applying lavender oil straight to the skin is normally harmless. You may also add around ten drops of lavender oil to a foot bath and revel in the relaxing smell and antimicrobial properties. If you have low blood pressure, lavender essential oil is not recommended for your feet.

Lemon Essential Oil: This is a 100% natural substance that can potentially be used as a home care cure. It's produced from fresh lemon peels using a cold-pressing technique that pricks and twists the peel while the oil is released. Many people mistake lemon essential oil for lemongrass essential oil, but the two are not the same. Lemon essential oil is derived from the citrus Lemon plant and used in aromatherapy. For a delightful scent, add a drop or two of diluted lemon essential oil to your bath and soak your feet. Lemon essential oil might help you feel less stressed and exhausted. Lemon essential oil can be diluted and applied directly on the skin, or it can be diffused and inhaled. Lemon essential oil is an anti-exhaustion, anti-depression, skin-clearing, anti-viral, anti-bacterial, anti-inflammatory, and anti-viral component. Lemon essential oil can assist to brighten dull skin and treat a variety of skin problems, including athlete's foot. Lemon essential oil should be used in a diluted form. It can be mixed with a carrier oil like avocado or jojoba.

Tea Tree Essential Oil: This oil is a popular natural medicine for treating bacterial and fungal skin infections, avoiding infection, and aiding healing due to its germ-fighting characteristics. Tea Tree essential oil is extracted from the leaves of Melaleuca Alternifolia, a tiny tree native to Australia. The antifungal and antibacterial effects of tea tree oil are well-known. It energizes both your mind and body. Tea tree oil may aid in the control of odour and the killing of microorganisms produced by perspiration. Tea tree oil is a natural alternative to antiperspirants and deodorants because of its antibacterial qualities. Many people believe the stench comes from the sweat glands, but it is actually bacteria that thrive on sweat. Sweat gland secretions produce a mild to strong odour when they come into touch with germs.

Grapefruit Essential Oil: This is derived from the glands found in the skin of the grapefruit. Grapefruit essential oil is extracted from the grapefruit peel glands. It's a citrus-scented oil with an orange tinge. Grapefruit essential oil is known for its antimicrobial and antibacterial characteristics and is used in aromatherapy. Grapefruit essential oil offers unique qualities that may assist your health in a variety of ways, including lowering blood pressure and stress levels. Grapefruit essential oil has been shown in numerous tests to have the ability to fight dangerous bacteria such as Staphylococcus aureus and Enterococcus faecalis. Grapefruit is the most powerful oil in terms of antibacterial activities, according to research. You can get rid of the germs that thrive in your foot perspiration, which will help you get rid of the unpleasant odour.

Peppermint Essential Oil: The benefits of this oil cannot be overlooked. Peppermint oil has the power to cleanse and renew skin, which is one of its best qualities. Peppermint essential oil is derived from the leaves of the peppermint plant and has a wide range of applications. Another excellent essential oil for removing unpleasant foot odour is peppermint. It has a calming and energizing effect on both the mind and the body. You can get rid of the stink by adding two drops of peppermint essential oil to your bath or foot soak. It also fights bacteria, which is the source of the stench in the first place.

CONCLUSION

Smelly feet are a common condition that usually goes away on its own. It can, however, be a symptom of a medical issue. Making foot care a regular part of your hygiene routine is the key. Home therapies are normally quite effective, although your doctor may recommend stronger treatments in severe cases. Foot odour can rapidly make any environment uncomfortable, and having smelly shoes is both embarrassing and unsanitary.

Fix it: Wearing bare feet in shoes is not a good idea. Socks act as a moisture absorber and provide a necessary barrier. Also, try not to wear the same pair every day; instead, alternate as much as possible. Instead of retaining moisture on your feet, choose socks that absorb it. Thick, comfortable socks made of natural fibers or athletic socks are examples.

Stay Dry: Bacteria that live on your feet and in your shoes thrive in damp environments. Bacteria won't want to live on your feet if you keep them dry. After coming out of the shower, properly dry your feet. If your feet are clammy or wet, don't wear socks or shoes.

Essential oils: This comes in different flavours and is a fantastic option for getting rid of stinky shoes. Many essential oils on the market today are excellent in removing the stench from shoes. Whether you use tea tree oil, eucalyptus oil, or clove oil, the oils will help remove the bacteria-caused shoe odour.

Foot hygiene: Wash and dry your feet every day, and change your socks at least once a day, preferably wool or cotton rather than nylon. Keep your toenails short and clean, and use a foot file to remove any hard skin. When moist, hard skin can become mushy, providing an excellent environment for germs to thrive. Between your toes, wash your feet. Moisture and heat are trapped in the toes, providing the ideal environment for germs to proliferate.

www.ingramcontent.com/pod-product-compliance
Lightning Source LLC
Chambersburg PA
CBHW061550250726
48657CB00006B/2419